# Chill to Heal

## How Cold Plunging and Contrast Therapy Can Transform Your Health

Harmony Royce

# DEDICATION

To individuals who have the guts to question the current quo, accept discomfort, and look for healing in unusual places. I hope this book encourages you to push yourself beyond your comfort zone, explore new wellness frontiers, and uncover the transformative potential of contrast therapy and cold plunging.

This is for everyone who believes in the body's ability to heal itself and for those who are constantly working on bettering themselves.

# DISCLAIMER

This book's content is meant exclusively for educational purposes and should not be interpreted as medical advice. Even though the advantages of contrast therapy and cold plunging are discussed based on the data that is currently available, it is crucial to speak with a healthcare provider before starting any new wellness program, particularly if you are pregnant or have underlying medical concerns. Any negative consequences, harm, or health issues resulting from the application of the methods and advice included in this book are not the responsibility of the author or publisher.

Always put safety first, pay attention to your body, and move cautiously.

# CONTENTS

# ACKNOWLEDGMENTS

My sincere appreciation goes out to everyone who helped to make this book possible. I want to start by expressing my gratitude to my family and friends for their everlasting conviction in my vision, support, and encouragement. Throughout the writing process, their understanding and patience were crucial.

I owe a debt of gratitude to the scholars, practitioners, and specialists whose work has influenced this book. I and many others are still motivated to investigate the therapeutic advantages of cold plunging and contrast treatment by their unwavering commitment to doing so.

I appreciate your interest in and dedication to your health and wellness journey, readers. I believe the information presented here will help you become more empowered, transform, and have a closer relationship with your body.

Finally, I want to express my gratitude to my mentors, editors, and everyone else who helped make this project a reality by providing advice, comments, and helpful critiques.

I sincerely appreciate your support, which is reflected in this book.

# CHAPTER 1

## AN OVERVIEW OF COLD PLUNGING AND CONTRAST THERAPY

## 1.1 An Introduction to Cold Plunging

### The Meaning and Background of Cold Plunging

Immersing the body in cold water, usually between 10°C and 15°C (50°F and 59°F), is known as "cold plunging" and is used to promote a number of physical and psychological advantages. This is a centuries-old habit that was common in ancient societies, such as Nordic and Roman customs. Because they felt it encouraged health and energy, the Romans included cold water baths in their thermae (bathhouses). Nordic tribes embraced the revitalizing qualities of diving into frozen lakes or fjords and used freezing waters to recuperate from strenuous physical exercises.

Cold plunging has become a vital component of wellness regimens in the modern era, especially for athletes, biohackers, and health aficionados. Its simplicity and wide-ranging benefits, which include lowering inflammation and increasing mental toughness, are what make it so appealing.

**The History of Contrast Treatment**

The practice of switching between heat and cold exposures, known as contrast therapy, has historical roots as well. Saunas and freezing lakes or snow were alternated in ancient Finnish and Russian societies. Utilizing the body's innate reactions to temperature fluctuations was intended to encourage relaxation, cleansing, and circulation.

Long before contemporary science started to disentangle the mechanics underlying the body's thriving response to dynamic stimuli, this dual-temperature technique represents an intuitive knowledge of that relationship.

# The Modern Wellness Culture's Growing Interest in These Practices

A greater emphasis on holistic health and performance optimization has led to a resurgence of cold plunging and contrast therapy in recent decades. These approaches have gained popularity because of proponents like Wim Hof, sometimes known as the "Iceman," who combined controlled breathing techniques with cold exposure. These methods are now part of popular wellness programs after being further verified by scientific research and social media platforms.

Their comeback is in line with a cultural trend toward natural, non-invasive methods of enhancing mental and physical well-being that prioritize healing and resilience.

## 1.2 Cold Exposure Mechanisms

### The Physiological Mechanisms of Cold Plunging

A series of physiological reactions are triggered by cold

plunging, which aids in the body's stress adaptation. The body immediately experiences vasoconstriction—the narrowing of blood vessels to save heat—when submerged in cold water. In addition to providing special health advantages including enhanced circulation and cardiovascular efficiency, this rerouting of blood flow toward essential organs guarantees life in cold temperatures.

Furthermore, brown adipose tissue (BAT), a kind of fat that produces heat by burning calories, is activated by cold plunge. This thermogenic impact has been connected to better metabolic function and aids in controlling body temperature.

**Thermoregulation's Science and Effects on the Body**

The body's capacity to keep its core temperature within a specific range in spite of outside influences is known as thermoregulation. This system is put to the test by cold exposure, which causes the body to release hormones and shiver.

**Important physiological reactions consist of:**

Norepinephrine is a hormone that improves mood, alertness, and focus.

- **Inflammation reduction:** Pro-inflammatory cytokine production is reduced by cold exposure, which facilitates recuperation from exercise or injury.

- **Improved immunological response:** Short-term exposure to cold stress has been demonstrated to boost white blood cell production, strengthening the immune system.

A potent therapeutic tool for both immediate recovery and long-term health optimization is produced by these effects taken together.

**The Autonomic Nervous System's Function in Cold Exposure**

An important factor in cold plunging is the autonomic nerve system (ANS), which controls involuntary body processes like digestion and heart rate. The sympathetic branch The ANS, also known as the "fight or flight" system, is activated by exposure to cold water. An adrenaline rush brought on by this activation increases energy and focus.

Repeated exposure to cold over time can strengthen the ANS's parasympathetic branch, which controls rest and recuperation. The body's ability to withstand stress is enhanced by this equilibrium between activity and relaxation, which also promotes general wellbeing.

## 1.3 Contrast Treatment: Two Methods

## Overview of Contrast Therapy and Its Fundamentals

In order to produce a dynamic recuperation experience, contrast therapy alternates between exposure to heat and cold. The idea is straightforward: cold constricts blood vessels, lowering inflammation and pain, while heat dilates them, enhancing circulation and muscle relaxation. Contrast treatment enhances each of these opposing forces by mixing them.

By producing a "vascular workout," the cycle of dilation and constriction improves blood flow and nutrition delivery to tissues while hastening the elimination of waste materials like lactic acid. Because of this, it works especially well for preventing injuries and promoting muscle recovery.

## How Changing from Hot to Cold Can Optimize Therapeutic Advantages

In ways that static therapies cannot, the interaction of hot and cold temperatures stimulates the neurological and circulatory systems. Among the main advantages are:

- **Improved muscle recovery**: The alternating temperatures speed up muscle healing by improving oxygen and nutrient delivery.

- **Pain relief**: Heat relieves tense muscles and cold lowers swelling, providing all-encompassing pain treatment.

- **Reduction of stress:** The autonomic nervous system is regulated by the opposing sensations, which encourage emotional equilibrium and relaxation.

A standard treatment can include two to three cycles of 10 to 15 minutes in a sauna or hot tub, followed by 2 to 5 minutes in an ice bath. By using this technique, the body is certain to benefit from both the calming effects of heat and the energizing impacts of cold.

## Common Contrast Therapy Practices: Hot Tubs, Ice Baths, and Saunas

Contrast therapy is adaptable and can be customized to meet the needs of each patient. Typical procedures consist of:

- **Saunas:** Sweating, cleansing, and relaxation are all encouraged by dry heat. Popular choices include Finnish saunas, which are frequently combined with chilly lakes or showers.

- **Ice baths:** Ice baths, a mainstay of cold exposure, are useful for improving healing and easing muscular stiffness.

- **Hot tubs**: These offer a milder type of heat exposure that is perfect for easing joint discomfort and relaxing muscles.

These components work together to produce a comprehensive approach to wellness that combines traditional wisdom with contemporary scientific knowledge.

Cold plunging and contrast therapy are examples of how modern science and age-old customs may coexist. These exercises are vital components of the contemporary wellness toolkit because they not only test the body's ability to cope with stress but also offer a route to better physical and mental health.

# CHAPTER 2

## The Science of Cold Plunging

## 2.1 The Body's Reactions to Immersion in Cold Water

**Blood Flow Dynamics and Vasoconstriction**

Immersion in cold water causes a physiological response known as vasoconstriction, in which blood vessels constrict to reduce heat loss. By ensuring that blood is diverted from the extremities to the essential organs, this reaction helps to maintain the body's core temperature. There are various advantages to this brief blood redistribution:

- **Improved circulation:** Vasodilation, or the dilation of blood vessels, occurs when the body leaves a cold environment. This allows oxygen-rich blood to surge back into tissues, aiding in healing and recovery.
- **Enhanced vascular tone**: Frequent exposure to cold

strengthens blood vessel walls, increasing their flexibility and lowering the likelihood of circulation problems like hypertension.

Cold plunging is a great exercise for cardiovascular health because of this mechanism, which is similar to a "vascular workout."

**Brown Fat Activation and Its Impact on Metabolism**

In contrast to white fat, which stores energy, brown adipose tissue (BAT) uses a mechanism known as thermogenesis to burn energy and produce heat. BAT is activated by cold exposure, which starts metabolic processes that:

- **Burn calories:** BAT activation may help control weight by raising energy expenditure.
- Control your blood sugar levels: Brown fat activation may aid in the management of metabolic diseases like diabetes by enhancing insulin sensitivity.

Recent findings indicate that frequent cold plunging may

increase the body's capacity to transform white fat into brown fat, which is metabolically active and thermogenic.

## Hormonal Changes: Endorphins, Cortisol, and Norepinephrine

Important hormones involved in mood regulation and stress management are released in response to cold plunges:

- **Norepinephrine:** A spike in norepinephrine occurs when submerged in cold water. This neurotransmitter lowers inflammation in the body while boosting energy, focus, and attention.
- Endorphins: Endorphins, sometimes known as "feel-good hormones," are released when you're exposed to cold and foster feelings of happiness and contentment.
- **Cortisol:** Regular practice has been demonstrated to enhance the body's stress-response mechanism, which may eventually lower baseline cortisol levels, even though the stress of cold exposure may cause cortisol levels to rise initially.

Together, these hormonal changes provide cold plunging its energizing and stress-relieving properties.

## 2.2 Modulation of the Immune System

## The Benefits of Cold Exposure on Immune Function

The immune system is profoundly affected by cold plunge. Immunity is strengthened by adaptive changes triggered by the physiological stress of cold immersion. Important mechanisms consist of:

- The vasoconstriction-vasodilation cycle enhances the distribution of immune cells to regions that require them the most, resulting in improved circulation.
- **Activation of stress proteins:** Heat-shock and cold-shock proteins, which strengthen the immune system and protect cells, are released in response to cold stress.

The body becomes more resistant to sickness as a result of

these changes, especially during the cold and flu seasons.

## The Connection Between White Blood Cell Production and Cold Exposure

Immersion in cold water has been associated with a higher generation of leukocytes (white blood cells), which are vital for the fight against infections. Frequent exposure strengthens the immune system's ability to fight off threats by:

- Increasing natural killer (NK) cell activity, which targets and eliminates malignant or contaminated cells.
- Increasing the generation of lymphocytes and monocytes, which are essential parts of the body's defense mechanism.

According to research, people who regularly engage in cold plunging have a lower risk of developing upper respiratory infections and may recuperate more quickly from those that do occur.

# Current Research on Cold Plunging's Impact on Infection Resistance and Inflammation

According to scientific research, exposure to colds can help lower chronic inflammation, which is a major contributor to a number of illnesses. For instance:

- **Decreased pro-inflammatory cytokines:** Systemic inflammation is decreased by cold plunging, which lowers levels of cytokines such as TNF-alpha and interleukin-6.
- **Increased anti-inflammatory response:** It encourages the release of the anti-inflammatory molecule interleukin-10.

According to these results, cold plunging may be used in conjunction with other therapies for inflammatory diseases such as arthritis and autoimmune illnesses.

## 2.3 Mental Health Impact

## Using Cold Exposure to Reduce Stress

An efficient and natural method of lowering stress is cold plunging. The sympathetic nervous system is triggered by the shock of cold immersion, resulting in an instantaneous release of norepinephrine and adrenaline, which:

Enhances general stress tolerance and builds resilience by teaching the body to adjust to controlled stress. It also raises heart rate and oxygen intake, which heightens attentiveness.

Regular exposure to cold gradually aids in autonomic nervous system regulation, bringing the body closer to equilibrium and lowering chronic stress.

**The Potential of Cold Plunging to Reduce Anxiety and Depressive Symptoms**

Research on the mood-boosting benefits of cold plunge is growing. Important mechanisms consist of:

- **Endorphin release:** As previously stated, exposure to cold causes endorphins to be released, which results in emotions of joy and bliss.

- **Decrease in inflammatory markers:** Depression has been associated with chronic inflammation. By treating this underlying reason, the anti-inflammatory properties of cold plunge may help reduce depression symptoms.

- **Increased resilience:** People frequently report feeling more confident and accomplished after enduring the discomfort of cold immersion on a regular basis.

According to some research, cold water therapy may potentially be used as an additional non-pharmaceutical treatment for sadness and anxiety.

## Scientific Studies Examining the Effects of Cold Water Therapy on Neurotransmitters

By altering neurotransmitter activity, cold plunging has a direct impact on brain chemistry. Important conclusions include:

- **Dopamine boost:** Dopamine levels can rise by up to 250% when exposed to cold water, which enhances motivation, concentration, and enjoyment.

- **Regulation of serotonin:** Exposure to cold promotes serotonin equilibrium, which is essential for emotional health.
- **Activity of beta-endorphin:** By interacting with the opioid receptors in the brain, these neuropeptides improve mood and lessen pain perception.

Because of these alterations in brain chemistry, cold plunging is an effective technique for enhancing emotional stability and mental clarity.

Cold plunging has a strong scientific foundation and is more than just a passing wellness fad. We discover its potential as a transformative practice for improving both physical and emotional well-being by investigating its benefits for the immune system, the body, and the mind.

# CHAPTER 3

## Cold Plunging's Therapeutic Advantages

### 3.1 Muscle Repair and Recuperation

### How Cold Plunging Aids in the Recovery of Athletes Following Vigorous Exercise

A vital component of recovery regimens for athletes in all sports is cold plunging. The technique speeds up muscle repair and lessens post-exercise weariness, which aids in recovery. Important mechanisms consist of:

- **Decrease in metabolic activity:** Immersion in cold water slows down the metabolism of muscle tissue, which lessens the accumulation of metabolic waste products such lactic acid that cause discomfort in the muscles.

- **Enhanced oxygenation:** The cycle of vasoconstriction and vasodilation guarantees effective elimination of waste materials and restores oxygen and nutrients to worn-out muscles.

Cold plunging is frequently used into training regimens by athletes to preserve optimal performance and minimize recovery time from injury or muscle strain.

## How Cold Therapy Helps Reduce Inflammation and Muscle Soreness

By reducing inflammation, cold plunging helps to prevent delayed onset muscular soreness (DOMS). After being submerged in cold water:

- In particular, pro-inflammatory cytokines are reduced, which suppresses inflammatory pathways.
- Temporarily limiting blood flow helps to reduce swelling in overused muscles.

Athletes can speed up recovery and avoid chronic injuries by alternating between rest and cold plunging, which reduces inflammation.

**Studies on the Benefits of Cold Plunging for Post-Exercise Recovery**

Cold plunging is effective for post-exercise recovery, according to an increasing amount of research. Among the noteworthy discoveries are:

- Up to 96 hours following vigorous activity, cold water immersion dramatically lessens muscular soreness, according to a 2016 meta-analysis that was published in the Journal of Sports Medicine.
- By speeding up recovery, research on top athletes has demonstrated that cold plunging helps sustain performance levels over the course of multiple training sessions or games.

Its usefulness in acute recovery situations is widely accepted, but its application for long-term muscle adaptation is up for debate.

## 3.2 Loss of Weight and Fat

Brown Adipose Tissue's Contribution to Cold-Induced Fat

Burning

BAT, or brown adipose tissue, is essential for cold-induced thermogenesis. In the presence of cold:

- **BAT is activated**, producing heat and regulating body temperature by burning calories. This process promotes energy expenditure and fat reduction in addition to helping with thermoregulation.

- Cold plunging is a potential weight-management technique since people with higher levels of active BAT may have better calorie-burning benefits.

## The Effects of Cold Exposure on Calorie Consumption and Metabolism

The body's ability to burn calories is increased when metabolic processes are stimulated by cold plunge. Important impacts consist of:

- Frequent exposure to cold enhances basal energy expenditure, even when at rest. This results in an increased resting metabolic rate (RMR).

- **Improved insulin sensitivity:** Exposure to cold improves glucose metabolism, which may eventually aid in lowering fat storage.

Because of these benefits, cold plunging is a useful complement to a more comprehensive weight loss or metabolic health plan.

## Proof of a Connection Between Weight Loss and Cold Plunging, Including Current Clinical Studies

Cold plunging and weight management are related, according to recent research:

- Depending on the length and degree of exposure, regular cold exposure can raise calorie expenditure by 15–30%, according to a 2014 study published in the Journal of Clinical Investigation.
- Clinical trials in 2022 showed that, in comparison to a control group, those who engaged in cold plunging three times a week for eight weeks saw a significant decrease in their body fat percentages.

Although cold plunging by itself is not a panacea, its metabolic advantages can enhance the benefits of a balanced diet and regular exercise.

## 3.3 Better Cardiovascular and Circulatory Health

**How Exposure to Cold Enhances Cardiovascular Health and Blood Flow**

As a vascular workout, cold plunging enhances circulation and blood flow. Submersion in cold water results in:

- Vasoconstriction: In order to preserve heat, blood vessels contract, which lowers blood flow to the extremities.
- Vasodilation: Blood vessels enlarge as a result of leaving a chilly environment, boosting the amount of oxygen-rich blood that reaches tissues.

By strengthening the vascular system, this cycle raises cardiovascular flexibility and efficiency.

**Regular Cold Plunging's Impact on Heart Rate**

**Variability (HRV)**

One important measure of the health of the cardiovascular and autonomic nerve systems is heart rate variability (HRV). HRV is positively impacted by cold plunging by:

- Increasing parasympathetic (rest-and-digest) activity, which balances the sympathetic dominance brought on by stress.
- Enhancing overall resilience via enhancing the heart's capacity to adjust to shocks.

Frequent cold plunge participants frequently report higher HRV scores, a metric linked to a lower risk of heart disease, better stress management, and longer lifespans.

**The Potential of Cold Therapy to Lower the Risk of Cardiovascular Conditions**

Cold plunging has the potential to lower the incidence of cardiovascular illnesses by increasing vascular health, decreasing inflammation, and boosting circulation. Important advantages include:

- **Decreased blood pressure:** Exposure to cold fosters healthy blood pressure management by teaching blood vessels to dilate and contract effectively.

- **Decreased arterial stiffness:** Research indicates that frequent cold plunges may enhance arterial flexibility, which is important in avoiding diseases like atherosclerosis.

- **Anti-inflammatory properties:** The capacity of cold plunging to reduce systemic inflammation adds a protective layer because chronic inflammation is a major factor to cardiovascular illnesses.

Early research indicates that including cold therapy in wellness routines may greatly improve cardiovascular health and longevity, but further long-term studies are required.

Numerous therapeutic advantages of cold plunging include enhanced cardiovascular function and quicker muscular regeneration. People can fully utilize this technique as part of an all-encompassing wellness approach by comprehending the underlying mechanics and using it effectively.

# CHAPTER 4

## THE COGNITIVE AND PSYCHOLOGICAL ADVANTAGES OF COLD PLUNGING

## 4.1 Resilience and Mental Toughness

### Regular Cold Plunging's Effect on Mental Hardiness

A significant mental workout that develops mental toughness, cold plunging is more than simply a physical activity. The natural reaction to discomfort must be overcome in order to submerge oneself in ice water, which:

- By educating the mind to persevere in trying circumstances, it strengthens willpower.
- The cultivation of a growth mindset is encouraged as practitioners get used to overcoming mental obstacles.
- Tolerance for discomfort is developed, which is a skill that helps one deal with hardship in day-to-day

life.

People are conditioned to venture outside of their comfort zones by cold plunging, which supports the notion that enduring regulated stress promotes human development.

**How Exposure to Cold Increases Emotional and Physical Stress Resilience**

Similar to how the body reacts to stress, cold immersion triggers the sympathetic nervous system. Regular exposure to cold over time:

- Enhances resilience by teaching the body and mind to bounce back from stress faster.
- The hypothalamic-pituitary-adrenal (HPA) axis is rebalanced, which enhances the body's responsiveness to stressors and lessens overreactions to small stimuli.

Because cold plunging involves maintaining composure and concentration while experiencing discomfort, it also promotes emotional regulation, which is a skill that may be applied to handling emotional difficulties.

## Perspectives on Cold Immersion Techniques from Psychological Research

The following research provide insight into the psychological advantages of exposure to cold:

- Regular cold exposure practice increased stress resilience and decreased burnout, according to a 2018 study published in the Journal of Psychology and Health.
- Cold immersion exercises have been shown to increase stress tolerance, improve psychological adaptation, and improve decision-making under pressure in military personnel.

These results support the benefits of regular cold plunging for mental toughness.

## 4.2 Increased Neurotransmitter Release and Mood

The Benefits of Cold Plunging for Elevating Dopamine

and Serotonin

Immersion in cold water sets off a series of neurochemical reactions that have a direct impact on emotional health and mood. In particular:

- dopamine, sometimes known as the "feel-good" neurotransmitter, is stimulated by cold plunging. A long-lasting feeling of motivation and pleasure is produced by this increase in dopamine levels.
- Additionally, serotonin levels are raised, which encourages calmness and lowers anxiety.
- Significant levels of norepinephrine, a hormone and neurotransmitter linked to energy and alertness, are produced, giving rise to an instant mood lift.

## The Connection Between Mood Elevation and Cold Exposure

The vagus nerve, which is essential for controlling mood and mental states, is activated by the sudden shock of cold water. This activation results in:

- A reduction in stress chemicals, especially cortisol,

which has a relaxing effect.

- Post-immersion bliss is a result of an increase in endorphins, the body's natural painkillers.

Many practitioners describe the technique as a mental "reset" and experience long-lasting improvements in their mood and mental clarity.

## The Potential of Cold Plunging to Treat Seasonal Affective Disorder (SAD)

Cold plunge may help those with Seasonal Affective Disorder, which is characterized by depression symptoms during the darker months. The procedure:

- By raising norepinephrine and dopamine levels, it combats sluggishness and low energy. It offers a simple and natural way to boost alertness and motivation during times when there is less sunlight.
- Anecdotal research suggests that it is effective in elevating mood and lowering depressed symptoms, and it has been incorporated into alternative therapy for SAD.

According to ongoing research, cold plunging may be used in addition to light therapy and medicine, which are conventional therapies for SAD.

## 4.3 Cognitive Function, Clarity, and Focus

## How Alertness and Mental Clarity Are Enhanced by Cold Plunging

The body's sympathetic nervous system is triggered by the physiological shock of cold immersion, leading to:

- As blood rushes to the brain and center, there is an increase in energy and alertness.
- the release of norepinephrine, which improves concentration and mental focus.
- a cerebral "wake-up" impact that can improve decision-making and productivity for hours following the fall.

Frequent users frequently claim increased mental clarity, characterizing the practice as a "mind-clearing" exercise that helps them fight off brain fog.

## The Possible Advantages of Cold Exposure for Concentration and Focus

Long-term cognitive advantages, namely in improving mental stamina and sustained attention, have been associated with exposure to cold. This is accomplished by:

- The brain is better oxygenated because of improved circulation. Neurogenesis, or the production of new brain cells, is stimulated, especially in areas related to memory and focus.

- Professionals, students, and anybody else looking for a mental advantage can all benefit from cold plunging since it can also help refocus focus.

## Scientific Data Examining the Effects of Cold Therapy on Brain Health

Recent studies highlight the neuroprotective advantages of exposure to cold:

- Regular exposure to colds may lower the risk of neurodegenerative diseases by raising brain-derived neurotrophic factor (BDNF) levels, according to a 2020 study published in Frontiers in Neuroscience.
- According to clinical studies, cold therapy can enhance executive function, which encompasses emotional control, decision-making, and planning.

Furthermore, exposure to cold enhances the brain's capacity to control stress-induced inflammation, which is essential for halting cognitive deterioration.

From strengthening mental toughness to elevating mood and concentration, cold plunging provides significant psychological and cognitive advantages. People can access both short-term and long-term mental health benefits by being aware of these impacts and including cold therapy into a well-rounded wellness regimen.

# CHAPTER 5

CONTRAST THERAPY: USING CHANGING TEMPERATURES TO OPTIMIZE HEALTH BENEFITS

## 5.1 Contrast Therapy Principles and Practice

## Comprehending the Changing Hot and Cold Method

In order to stimulate the body's physiological systems, contrast treatment strategically alternates heat and cold exposures. The idea is to use heat stress to provide a regulated shock that strengthens the body's defenses against injury and deterioration.

- **Hot exposure** (such as saunas and hot baths) causes vasodilation, which increases blood flow, relaxes muscles, and encourages sweating, which aids in cleansing.
- Vasoconstriction brought on by cold exposure (ice baths, cold showers, etc.) lowers inflammation,

increases circulation, and improves mental clarity. By switching between these extremes, the body is trained to adjust swiftly, which enhances physical performance and general stress resilience.

The technique has its origins in antiquated customs that highlighted the benefits of thermal fluctuation for health and longevity, such as the Scandinavian sauna culture and hydrotherapy in traditional medicine.

**Typical Contrast Treatment Procedures**

It is possible to modify contrast therapy to suit each patient's requirements and preferences. Typical techniques consist of:

- **Hot/Cold Showers:** For multiple cycles, alternate between two to three minutes of warm water and thirty to one minute of cold water.
- **Ice Bath/Sauna Combinations:** repeatedly immerse yourself in an ice bath for 1–5 minutes after spending 10–20 minutes in a sauna.
- **Hydrotherapy Pools:** These pools alternate between

hot and cold water to safely and efficiently promote temperature changes.

## The Advantages of Changing Temperatures for Relaxation and Muscle Recovery

In contrast therapy, the interaction of heat and cold provides a potent blend of relaxation and recuperation advantages:

- **Muscle Recovery:** Changing temperatures speeds up tissue healing, lessens post-exercise muscle discomfort, and aids in the removal of metabolic waste.
- **Relaxation:** A balanced feeling of peace and renewal is left after the hot phase relieves stress and the cold phase energizes.

In order to sustain optimal performance, contrast treatment is frequently a crucial part of rehabilitation regimens for athletes and health lovers.

## 5.2 Nervous System Impacts

## How Contrast Therapy Affects Sympathetic and Parasympathetic System Stimulation

By activating both autonomic nervous system branches, contrast treatment provides a well-rounded method of relaxation and recuperation:

- **Sympathetic Activation:** The fight-or-flight response is triggered by the cold phase, which increases alertness by promoting the release of norepinephrine.
- **Parasympathetic Activation:** The heat phase promotes relaxation and lowers stress hormones by boosting rest-and-digest processes.

After experiencing physical or emotional stress, this dual activation helps the body regain homeostasis by recalibrating the neural system.

## The Impact of Changing Temperatures on the

## Autonomic Nervous System

The neurological system gets a dynamic "workout" from the temperature changes:

- Exposure to cold improves thermoregulation, which teaches the body to adjust to environmental stimuli more effectively.
- In order to maintain blood vessels' flexibility and responsiveness, hot exposure enhances vascular compliance.
- When combined, they train the nervous system to better handle stress on the body and mind.

Better resilience, a quicker recovery from stressors, and an increased sense of general well-being can all be outcomes of this adaptation.

## Using Contrast Therapy to Improve Relaxation and Recovery

Recovery is improved by the precisely timed transition between hot and cold phases because:

- Enhancing circulation and eliminating contaminants.
- Reducing muscular and joint swelling and inflammation.
- By regulating the neurological system, deep relaxation is encouraged.

For people recovering from strenuous exercise, managing chronic pain, or coping with stress-related problems, contrast treatment is especially beneficial.

## 5.3 Improved Circulation and Detoxification

## How Contrast Therapy Promotes Lymphatic Drainage and Detoxification

Sweating, a natural detoxification process that aids in the removal of toxins such heavy metals and metabolic waste products, is induced during the heat phase of contrast therapy. Exposure to cold, in turn:

- Promotes lymphatic circulation, which helps flush out extra fluid and cellular debris.
- Promotes deep breathing, which improves oxygen

exchange and CO2 removal, thereby aiding detoxification.

When combined, these benefits maximize the body's natural detoxification processes, leaving people feeling renewed and invigorated.

## The Advantages of Better Tissue Circulation and Oxygenation

Because of the cyclical expansion and contraction of blood vessels, contrast treatment dramatically improves circulation:

- Increased blood flow from heat-induced vasodilation helps tissues get nutrients and oxygen while eliminating waste.
- Vasoconstriction brought on by cold concentrates blood flow to essential organs and returns a surge of oxygenated blood to peripheral tissues as the body warms up.

This dynamic mechanism accelerates the healing of

worn-out or damaged tissues and improves cardiovascular health overall.

## Studies on the Potential of Contrast Therapy to Lower Toxins and Encourage Healing

Research demonstrates the therapeutic and cleansing effects of contrast therapy:

- According to a 2019 study published in the Journal of Athletic Recovery, athletes who received contrast therapy had better lymphatic function and less inflammatory markers.
- Regular contrast treatment sessions were found to significantly increase endothelial function and blood flow, according to research published in Circulatory Health.
- Practitioners' anecdotal evidence emphasizes the therapy's potential to treat ailments like poor circulation, persistent pain, and arthritis.

Contrast therapy is a potent tool for attaining holistic health and wellness since it improves the body's capacity for detoxification and healing.

By combining hot and cold exposure, contrast treatment provides a synergistic method to optimize health advantages. It has enormous potential for both physical and mental healing, from enhancing circulation and cleansing to controlling the neurological system. A new depth of health and vigor can be unlocked by incorporating contrast treatment into a routine, whether it be through basic hot/cold showers or more sophisticated sauna and ice bath routines.

# CHAPTER 6

## IMMUNE SYSTEM SUPPORT AND COLD PLUNGING

## 6.1 Cold Exposure Activates the Immune System

### How the Immune System Is Activated by Cold Plunging

The body's innate and adaptive immunological responses are triggered by cold plunge, preparing it to fight off infections more successfully. Cold exposure triggers a regulated stress response in the body that fortifies immune response and surveillance systems.

- The stress hormone norepinephrine, which has been demonstrated to lower inflammation and boost immune function, is produced in response to the shock of cold exposure.
- The hypothalamic-pituitary-adrenal (HPA) axis is also activated by this cold-induced stress, which regulates immunological function and aids in the

body's adaptation to environmental changes.

## The physiological mechanism that triggers the production of cytokines and white blood cells

Exposure to cold enhances immunological activity by:

- **Increasing white blood cell activity:** The body's defenses against infections are strengthened by the mobilization of leukocytes, or white blood cells, brought on by the brief stress of cold plunge.
- **Stimulating cytokine production:** Pro-inflammatory cytokines including TNF-alpha and IL-6, which function as signaling molecules to attract immune cells during acute stressors, are elevated in response to cold immersion. This eventually results in improved inflammation control.

## Studies Illustrating How Cold Therapy Affects Immune Response

Numerous studies have shown how exposure to cold can strengthen the immune system:

- Regular cold-water immersion increased leukocyte and natural killer (NK) cell counts, which are critical for fighting cancers and viruses, according to a study published in PLOS One.

- Interleukin-6 (IL-6), which promotes tissue regeneration and acute immunological response, was shown to be higher among cold-water swimmers, according to research published in Frontiers in Physiology.

- The Wim Hof Method has demonstrated promise in lowering inflammatory responses and enhancing resistance to pathogens introduced in experiments by combining breathing techniques with cold exposure.

## 6.2 Recovery and Inflammation

## Cold Therapy's Contribution to Lowering Systemic Inflammation

Numerous illnesses, such as metabolic syndromes, autoimmune diseases, and cardiovascular ailments, are significantly influenced by chronic inflammation. The way cold plunging reduces inflammation is by:

- Inflamed tissues receive less blood flow, which lessens swelling and irritation.
- In order to control inflammation and maintain metabolic health, anti-inflammatory molecules like adiponectin are released.
- Improving the lymphatic system, which helps tissues rid themselves of waste and inflammatory mediators.

## The Benefits of Cold Plunging for Inflammatory Disease Recovery

It is commonly known that cold therapy works well for reducing inflammation brought on by both acute traumas and long-term illnesses:

- Cold plunging is a typical technique used by athletes to treat exercise-induced inflammation, which speeds up recovery by lowering joint swelling and muscle soreness.
- The potential of cold therapy to relieve pain and stiffness is beneficial for chronic inflammatory

disorders including tendinitis and arthritis.

## Using Cold Plunging to Treat Chronic Inflammation and Autoimmune Diseases

In autoimmune diseases like lupus or rheumatoid arthritis, the body's tissues are attacked by the immune system. Cold plunging is not a remedy, but it can:

- Reduce inflammatory indicators, such as C-reactive protein (CRP), which are frequently raised in autoimmune diseases.
- Reduce pain, swelling, and exhaustion to alleviate symptoms.
- Enhance overall quality of life and assist control immunological activity to support other treatments.

New studies are still being conducted to investigate the potential supplementary advantages of cold exposure for those with chronic inflammatory diseases.

## 6.3 The Connection Between Immune Function and Mental Health

## Examining the Connection Between Mental Health and Immune Function

Researchers refer to this strong relationship between the immune system and mental health as the immune-brain axis. While a strong immune system promotes emotional resilience, long-term stress and mental illness can impair immunological defenses. In this dynamic, cold plunging contributes by:

- Adjusting stress hormones, such cortisol, which can affect immune function if they are dysregulated.
- Increasing the production of endorphins and dopamine, elevating mood, and lessening the detrimental effects of stress on immunity.

## The Impact of Cold Exposure on the Body's Immune Resilience and Stress Response

The acute stress response is triggered by cold plunging and

aids in the body's gradual adaptation to stressors:

- The stress-response system is strengthened by cold exposure, which enables the body to manage stress more skillfully without getting overstimulated.

- **Decreased chronic inflammation:** Cold plunging can help reduce the low-grade inflammation that is frequently linked to long-term stress by regulating immunological activity.

- **Better sleep**: Sleep is crucial for mental and immunological health, and cold plunging can improve the quality of your sleep.

## Findings from Continued Research on the Potential of Cold Plunging to Treat Stress and Depression

Research on mental health is beginning to focus on cold plunging because of its possible benefits as a treatment for stress and depression:

- According to a study published in Medical Hypotheses, submersion in cold water stimulates the parasympathetic nervous system, which promotes relaxation and lessens depressive symptoms.

- Psychoneuroendocrinology research revealed that exposure to cold raises dopamine and beta-endorphin levels, which are neurotransmitters associated with stress reduction and mood control.

- The long-term effects of cold plunging on stress resilience and its potential as a supplemental treatment for mood disorders are presently being examined in clinical trials.

By lowering inflammation and strengthening the vital link between immunity and mental health, cold plunging has significant positive effects on the immune system. Cold therapy is a holistic approach to boosting general health and wellbeing by promoting immunological activation, controlling systemic inflammation, and strengthening stress resilience. Cold plunge is a potent weapon in the toolbox of contemporary wellness, whether it is employed to increase mental clarity, manage chronic diseases, or aid in recovery.

# CHAPTER 7

### FAT LOSS AND COLD PLUNGING

In addition to its therapeutic and recuperative advantages, cold plunging has become known as a weight-management and fat-loss technique. This chapter explores how exposure to cold affects fat metabolism, increases calorie expenditure, and promotes long-term weight control.

## 7.1 Thermogenesis and Fat Burning Induced by Cold

## How Cold Exposure Affects Brown Fat Activation

Brown adipose tissue (BAT), often known as brown fat, is stimulated by cold plunging. Brown fat produces heat by burning calories, a process known as non-shivering thermogenesis, in contrast to white fat, which stores energy.

- **How it works:** The "powerhouses" of cells,

mitochondria, are found in great concentration in brown fat. BAT increases energy expenditure by activating to produce heat when exposed to cold.

- **Evolutionary significance:** This system is a useful tool for fat metabolism since it evolved to assist humans maintain core body temperature in cold situations.

## How Dropping in the Cold Increases Calorie Consumption

The body has to work harder to maintain homeostasis after the cold shock of immersion, which raises the basal metabolic rate (BMR):

- **Energy demand**: The sympathetic nervous system is triggered by cold exposure, which speeds up metabolic processes.
- **Sustained calorie burn:** Research indicates that when the body works to restore thermal balance, calorie expenditure may continue to rise for hours after submersion.

# Clinical Research Shows a Connection Between Cold Therapy and Fat Loss

An increasing amount of studies demonstrates how exposure to cold can aid in fat loss:

- According to a study in The Journal of Clinical Investigation, people who had higher levels of brown fat activity burnt a lot more calories when they were chilly.

- Regular exposure to cold can eventually result in quantifiable decreases in body fat, especially in areas with strong BAT activity, according to research published in Obesity Reviews.

- A 2020 study published in *Cell Metabolism* revealed that participants in controlled cold exposure regimens had decreased levels of white adipose tissue and increased fat metabolism.

## 7.2 The Study of Cold Adaptation

# The Physiologic Mechanism of Cold Exposure Adaptation

The body becomes more adept at using fat as an energy source as a result of physiological changes brought on by repeated exposure to cold conditions.

- Cold plunging gradually improves the body's capacity to activate brown fat and withstand lower temperatures without experiencing severe discomfort.
- **Thermal efficiency**: People who have adapted to cold have better thermogenic reactions, which results in steady calorie burning when exposed to cold.

## How Frequent Cold Plunging Boosts the Effectiveness of Fat Burning

**Adaptation to exposure to cold leads to:**

- **Enhanced mitochondrial function:** When brown fat is repeatedly activated, the quantity and effectiveness of mitochondria are increased, increasing total energy expenditure.
- **Improved lipid metabolism:** This helps the body

lose weight by improving its ability to break down stored fat to meet energy needs.

- **Change in energy pathways:** Even at rest or during low-intensity activities, exposure to cold promotes the use of fat as the main energy source.

## Impact of Cold Therapy on Insulin Sensitivity and Metabolic Rate

Exposure to cold has a beneficial effect on metabolic health:

- **Increased metabolic rate:** Research indicates that, depending on exposure time and intensity, cold plunging can increase BMR by as much as 30%.

- **Improved insulin sensitivity**: Insulin resistance, a major contributor to fat storage, is decreased by cold exposure. Cold plunging helps reduce belly fat and prevent weight gain by enhancing glucose metabolism.

- **Decreased inflammation:** Cold plunging indirectly promotes metabolic processes that are essential for fat loss by reducing systemic inflammation.

## 7.3 Weight Loss and Cold Plunging

## The Function of Cold Exposure in Long-Term Fat Loss and Weight Management

Cold plunging contributes significantly to long-term weight management even though it is not a stand-alone weight loss method:

- **Preventing fat regain:** Cold therapy helps prevent the typical problem of weight regain by enhancing insulin sensitivity and maintaining a greater metabolic rate.
- **Hormonal balance:** Exposure to cold reduces hunger and increases satiety by regulating hunger hormones such as ghrelin and leptin.

## Combining Exercise, Diet, and Cold Therapy for Best Outcomes

Cold plunging should be incorporated within an all-encompassing lifestyle strategy for optimal results:

- **Dietary considerations**: To promote muscle repair and fat reduction, combine cold plunging with a well-balanced diet full of whole foods and enough protein.

- **Work together:** As part of your post-workout recovery regimen, use cold plunging to sustain high energy expenditure and improve muscle repair.

- **Consistency:** Frequent exposure to cold increases its fat-burning effects and guarantees long-term benefits.

## An Analysis of Research on the Impact of Cold Therapy on Body Composition

Cold plunging has been shown in numerous research to improve body composition.

- According to a study published in Nature Metabolism, exposure to cold lowers visceral fat, which is strongly associated with metabolic disorders.

- A study published in The American Journal of

Clinical Nutrition revealed that people who added cold immersion to their routines lost more body fat than those who only used diet and exercise.

- According to Sports Medicine research, cold therapy helps athletes and active people maintain lean body mass during weight reduction stages.

One useful technique for improving fat metabolism and aiding in weight management is cold plunging. Cold therapy is a scientifically supported method of fat loss by promoting metabolic health, activating brown fat, and raising calorie expenditure. It provides a long-term route to reaching and preserving ideal body composition when paired with a healthy lifestyle. Cold plunging is a useful supplement to any fat loss plan, whether for its short-term effects on burning calories or its long-term advantages for metabolic efficiency.

# CHAPTER 8



SAFETY CONSIDERATIONS AND RISKS

Even though cold plunge has several health advantages, there are hazards involved. To guarantee a satisfying and secure experience, it is crucial to have a thorough awareness of the possible risks and to follow safety regulations. This chapter examines the dangers of cold plunging, offers practical safety advice, and emphasizes contrast therapy safety measures.

## 8.1 Possible Dangers of Freezing

**The Risks Associated with Cold Exposure: Shock, Cardiovascular Stress, and Hypothermia**

When done incorrectly, cold plunging exposes the body to extremely high temperatures, which might have negative consequences:

- Long-term exposure to cold water can result in hypothermia, a condition where body temperature falls below the acceptable range of 35°C or 95°F. If left untreated, the symptoms which include severe shivering, disorientation, and loss of coordination can worsen and become life-threatening.

- A sudden immersion in cold water can cause an involuntary gasp response, hyperventilation, or an elevated heart rate, which can cause cardiovascular stress or drowning in susceptible people.

- **Cardiovascular Risks:** The stress of rapid vasoconstriction (tightening of blood vessels) might result in arrhythmias, chest pain, or in extreme situations, heart attacks, in people with underlying heart disorders.

## How to Identify and Prevent Unfavorable Cold Plunge Reactions

**It's critical to keep an eye on how your body reacts to cold immersion:**

**Identifying warning signs:**

- Severe shivering or numbness that doesn't go away after getting out of the water.
- Breathing difficulties, disorientation, or dizziness.
- An irregular heartbeat or persistent chest discomfort.

**Preventive measures:**

- As your body adjusts, progressively extend exposure times from short first exposures.
- Start with partial exposure, like your hands or feet, rather than complete submersion at first.
- If you experience more pain or discomfort than you can handle, you should always get out of the water.

## The Value of Adapting to Cold Therapy Gradually

Extreme temperatures take time for the human body to adjust to:

- **Acclimatization process:** Your cardiovascular and neurological systems can adjust to cold exposure gradually, lowering your risk of stress or cold shock.
- Regular or daily short exposures are safer and more helpful than long plunges that are done infrequently.

- **Paying attention to your body:** Individuals adapt differently; the procedure should be guided by personal tolerance.

## 8.2 Cold Plunging Safety Instructions

## Safe Cold Plunging Best Practices, Including Temperature and Duration Guidelines

Adhering to evidence-based recommendations maximizes advantages and guarantees safety:

**Recommendations for temperature:**
- **For novices:** Temperature range for water: 10°C to 15°C (50°F to 59°F).
- For professionals with experience: Although temperatures as low as 4°C (39°F) could be bearable, they shouldn't be tried without first adjusting.

**Duration:**
- For novices, start with 30 seconds to 2 minutes.
- Work up to five to ten minutes gradually as your

tolerance increases.

- **Environment:** Make sure there is a regulated environment with quick access to warmth and help when required.

How to Determine Your Level of Preparedness for Cold Plunging A safe cold therapy session depends on preparation:

- **Health assessment**: If you have any pre-existing conditions, particularly respiratory or cardiovascular problems, see a doctor.
- Mental preparedness: To prevent stress brought on by panic, approach cold diving with composure and concentration.
- **Physical preparation:** Before submersion, perform mild warm-up activities to stabilize blood circulation.

**Important Safety Measures for Individuals with Comorbidities**

Some folks must be very cautious:

- **Cardiovascular conditions:** Cold plunging should not be done without a doctor's approval if a person has high blood pressure, arrhythmias, or recent cardiac events.

- **Respiratory issues**: Cold-induced hyperventilation can aggravate conditions such as asthma.

- **Neurological concerns:** People who have epilepsy or other illnesses involving the nerves may have negative consequences from cold immersion.

## 8.3 Controlling Contrast Therapy Risks

**Safety Issues When Using Cold and Hot Therapies Together**

There are particular difficulties with contrast therapy, which alternates between hot and cold:

- **Temperature extremes:** The cardiovascular system may be strained by abrupt changes from intense heat (saunas) to cold exposure.

- **Dehydration risk:** Heat exposure can cause fluid

loss, and if hydration is not maintained, this can make cold-induced stress worse.

- **Overexertion:** The body may get fatigued or experience extended stress as a result of repeated cycles of contrast therapy.

## Tips for a Secure Contrast Treatment Experience

A safe and efficient experience is guaranteed when best practices are followed:

- **Controlled transitions:** Give your body time to acclimate to periods of heat and cold. Before switching, let it settle at room temperature for a few minutes.
- **Hydration:** To compensate for fluid loss, drink water all during the workout.
- **Duration**: To prevent overstressing the body, limit the amount of time spent in each phase (cold or hot). Cycles typically last one to three minutes for cold and ten to fifteen minutes for hot.

## Suggestions for People with Respiratory or

## Cardiovascular Conditions

Contrast treatment must be used with caution in certain populations:

- **Cardiovascular health:** People with heart problems should stay away from sudden or drastic changes in temperature. Before starting contrast therapy, consult a doctor.

- **Respiratory issues:** To reduce cold shock or heat-induced hyperventilation, gradual exposure and breathing control are crucial.

- **Support and monitoring:** Always have someone close by to help out if necessary.

Although contrast treatment and cold plunging have revolutionary health benefits, safety precautions and hazards must be carefully considered. Practitioners can safely experience the restorative benefits of cold immersion while lowering risks by being aware of potential hazards, following best procedures, and customizing methods to meet the requirements of each individual. To ensure that these therapies are both safe and successful, preparation, gradual adaptation, and self-awareness should always come first.

# CHAPTER 9



TAKING A RISK IN THE CONTEMPORARY WELLNESS SECTOR

From a specialized activity to a vital component of the contemporary wellness sector, cold plunging has changed throughout time. Its growing importance is demonstrated by its integration into exercise, recuperation, and therapeutic regimens. The rise in popularity of cold plunging, its incorporation into exercise and recuperation regimens, and new developments influencing its future are all covered in this chapter.

## 9.1 How Common Cold Plunging Is at Spas and Wellness Facilities

**The Growth of Wellness Retreats Providing Contrast Therapy and Cold Plunging**

Cold plunging is becoming a staple of wellness spas' services all over the world:

- In order to offer a complete wellness package, luxury retreats and holistic health facilities frequently use cold immersion pools in addition to yoga, meditation, and sauna treatments.

- **Therapeutic focus:** Cold plunging sessions are advertised for its ability to enhance bodily regeneration, emotional resilience, and mental clarity.

## The Increasing Inclusion of Ice Baths in Spa Menus and Fitness Facilities

Cold therapy is becoming more widely available outside of upscale wellness facilities:

- **Spa inclusions:** To maximize relaxation and recuperation, massages and heat therapies are frequently paired with ice baths and cold therapy, which are now commonplace in spa menus.

- **Fitness centers:** Realizing the importance of cold therapy in improving workout performance and recuperation, several gyms now provide specialized cold therapy areas or equipment like portable ice baths.

## The Impact of Social Media and Celebrity Endorsements on Cold Plunging

Influencers and celebrities have been crucial in making cold plunging more widely accepted:

- **Endorsements:** Athletes, wellness advocates, and public personalities like Wim Hof frequently reveal their cold plunging regimens, giving the practice legitimacy and exposure.

- **Social media trends:** Viral videos promoting ice baths and their alleged health benefits are posted on platforms such as Instagram and TikTok, encouraging followers to follow suit.

- **Community engagement:** Online challenges, such "cold plunge challenges," encourage participation and spread the word about cold treatment to a variety of audiences.

## 9.2 Including Cold Plunging in Exercise and Recuperation Routines

## How Fitness Fanatics and Athletes Are Including Cold Therapy in Their Daily Routines

Cold treatment is used by athletes and fitness enthusiasts to enhance performance and recuperation:

- **Post-workout recovery:** After vigorous exercise, cold plunge speeds up recovery by reducing muscular discomfort.
- **Pre-event preparation:** Before a competition, some athletes use cold exposure to increase circulation and concentrate.

## Cold Plunging's Contribution to Injury Prevention and Healing

Cold therapy is essential for treating wounds and stopping additional harm:

- **Reducing inflammation:** Ice baths are frequently

used to reduce inflammation and swelling brought on by sports injuries.

- **Quicker recovery:** Recovery from small injuries is accelerated by cold exposure, which promotes blood flow and tissue restoration.
- **Pain management:** Following cold plunging sessions, athletes report feeling less pain, which increases their range of motion.

## Examples of Teams and Professional Athletes Using Cold Plunging

Elite athletes and sports teams around the world enjoy cold plunging:

- **Professional teams:** To guarantee the best player recuperation, rugby, basketball, and football teams incorporate cold immersion into their training plans.
- **Endurance athletes:** Cold treatment is used by triathletes and marathon runners to recuperate from the strain of extended physical activity.
- The use of cold treatment by Michael Phelps during his Olympic training is one of the more well-known

examples.

- LeBron James of the NBA uses ice baths as part of his strict recuperation regimen.

## 9.3 Upcoming Developments and Trends in Cold Plunging

**New Developments in Cold Therapy Technology, Such as Home Ice Bath Systems and Cryotherapy Chambers**

Cold therapy is becoming more effective and accessible thanks to technological advancements:

- **Cryotherapy chambers:** These cutting-edge devices provide regulated whole-body cooling, with short sessions reaching temperatures as low as -110°C (-166°F) to provide the benefits of cold therapy without complete submersion in water.
- **Portable ice baths:** Small and easy-to-use devices are becoming more and more popular for usage at home, allowing people to conveniently perform cold therapy.
- **Intelligent monitoring tools:** During cold plunging

sessions, innovations such as wearable technology monitor recovery parameters, heart rate, and temperature exposure.

## Contrast Therapy's Future and Its Significance for Contemporary Health and Wellbeing

Contrast treatment is becoming a more common therapeutic choice:

- **Integration with other therapies:** It is increasingly common for wellness programs that use cold plunging with hydrotherapy, physiotherapy, and infrared saunas.
- **Personalized protocols**: Individualized contrast therapy regimens are becoming more popular, depending on personal health indicators.
- **Corporate wellness programs:** To increase employee productivity and lower stress levels, employers are implementing cold therapy into workplace wellness programs.

## Continued Investigation into the Benefits of Cold

## Plunging for Different Medical Conditions

The possible uses of cold therapy are still being investigated by scientists:

- Research is looking into cold plunging as a non-invasive treatment for arthritis and fibromyalgia in cases of chronic pain.
- Research has shown that exposure to cold helps reduce symptoms of anxiety, depression, and post-traumatic stress disorder (PTSD).
- **Metabolic health:** Research is still being conducted to determine whether cold therapy can help people with metabolic disorders manage their weight and improve their insulin sensitivity.

Cold plunging's increasing popularity in the wellness sector is evidence of its transformational potential. Cold therapy is revolutionizing the contemporary approach to health and well-being through its incorporation into fitness and recuperation regimens and the use of cutting-edge technologies. Cold plunging is set to become an essential part of holistic wellness practices as further research confirms its advantages.

# CHAPTER 10

**T**HE **F**UTURE OF **C**OLD **P**LUNGING AND **C**ONTRAST **T**HERAPY: **C**URRENT **S**TUDIES AND **C**LINICAL **T**RIALS

The therapeutic technique of cold plunging appears to have a bright future as it continues to gain popularity in fitness circles, wellness centers, and spas. The current research, the possibility of mainstream medical integration, and the significance of public education on cold plunging and contrast therapy are all covered in detail in this chapter. We discuss the potential for these treatments to become a mainstay of healthcare, the ways in which clinical trials and developing research are revealing new advantages, and the growing significance of informing the public about their safe usage.

## 10.1 Important Research and Studies in 2024

## Summary of Current Cold Therapy Clinical Trials and Research

Numerous clinical trials are now being conducted to examine cold therapy, specifically through techniques like cold plunging and contrast therapy. Universities and research organizations are investing a lot of money in learning about the physiological and psychological impacts of exposure to cold:

- **Exploratory studies**: A number of clinical trials are being conducted to evaluate the therapeutic benefits of cold therapy for chronic diseases as well as its impact on recovery following physical exertion. Its potential to lower inflammation, hasten muscle repair, and improve general physical recovery is being studied.

- **Innovative applications:** Research is looking into how cold exposure might boost immune responses, treat mental health conditions, and improve cognitive function.

The results of these studies, which aim to give a more thorough understanding of the effects of cold plunge on human health, have the potential to completely alter our perspective on healing and well-being.

## Positive Results in the Domains of Immune Response, Mental Health, and Fat Loss

Promising findings are emerging from studies on the effects of cold therapy, particularly in the areas of immune system function, mental health, and weight loss:

- **Mental health:** Research has shown that exposure to cold may be beneficial for mood disorders like anxiety and depression. It has been demonstrated that cold plunging causes the release of norepinephrine, a neurotransmitter associated with elevated mood and mental acuity. According to research, exposure to cold may have antidepressant effects naturally by boosting circulation to important brain regions linked to emotional regulation and inducing the fight-or-flight response.

- **Immune function:** The function of cold plunging in immune support is one of the most interesting research topics. According to studies, cold therapy increases the body's defenses by activating white blood cells. Research on the effects of cold exposure on the immune system, sickness duration, and even chronic autoimmune disorders is still ongoing.

- **Fat loss:** Fat burning has been associated with cold-induced thermogenesis, the process by which the body produces heat to compensate for exposure to cold. According to new research, cold therapy may help people lose weight and reduce body fat by activating brown adipose tissue, or brown fat, which burns calories to generate heat. The usefulness of cold exposure as a supplement to diet and exercise for people seeking long-term fat loss is being investigated in recent studies.

## An Examination of Cold Therapy's Potential as a Chronic Illness Treatment

The possibility of cold plunging to cure chronic diseases is also being investigated:

- The potential of cold therapy as a treatment for inflammatory disorders such arthritis, fibromyalgia, and persistent back pain is being investigated in clinical trials. According to preliminary study, cold exposure reduces swelling and numbs nerve endings, which speeds up recovery and provides long-term pain relief.

- **Neurological disorders:** Research is looking into whether cold therapy can help control the symptoms of neurological conditions like Parkinson's disease or multiple sclerosis. By enhancing blood circulation and preserving neuronal integrity, cold exposure may lessen the symptoms of these disorders, which frequently cause inflammation or damage to the nervous system.

Cold therapy may prove to be a flexible and affordable treatment for a number of chronic illnesses when additional information from these studies becomes available.

## 10.2 Mainstream Medicine's Risk of Cold Plunging

## How Cold Therapy May Emerge as a Popular Choice for Mental Health and Physical Healing

Because of its proven benefits for immune system performance, muscular recovery, and mental health, cold therapy is becoming more and more popular in mainstream medicine:

- **Mental health:** Cold plunging may be suggested as a treatment for mood problems as a supplement to traditional therapy. Researchers are examining whether cold exposure could be a non-invasive, easily accessible solution for people at risk of anxiety or depression.

- **Physical recovery:** Cold treatment is already a mainstay for muscle rehabilitation among athletes and fitness aficionados. Cold plunging has been the preferred treatment due to the advantages of decreased inflammation and accelerated healing time frames. For patients recovering from surgery or undergoing physical rehabilitation, the medical community may implement cold therapy procedures, maybe as a component of a more comprehensive recovery plan.

Healthcare professionals may start including cold plunging and contrast treatment in recovery plans for patients with musculoskeletal injuries, arthritis, or even mental health issues as clinical data grows.

## The Possible Use of Contrast Therapy to Treat Chronic Conditions Like Arthritis or Fibromyalgia

Patients with chronic illnesses may benefit greatly from the introduction of contrast therapy, which alternates between hot and cold treatments, into mainstream medicine:

- **Fibromyalgia:** Patients who have this condition frequently report stiffness, exhaustion, and widespread muscle discomfort. According to certain research, contrast therapy which alternates between cold and heat may lessen the feeling of pain and enhance circulation, making it a useful tool for managing pain.

- Both hot and cold therapy have been used to help people with arthritis with their joint pain, stiffness, and swelling. A comprehensive strategy for controlling chronic pain can be achieved by alternating between hot and cold therapy, which can increase joint mobility and lower inflammation.

Contrast therapy may become a common treatment option in physical therapy clinics and chronic pain management facilities if additional research validates its advantages for these disorders.

## Including Cold Plunging in Medical Procedures for Holistic Care

Soon, cold plunging may be used in integrative medicine procedures, which mix it with other therapies to provide a comprehensive approach to health:

- **Complementary therapy:** Cold plunging is a non-invasive, drug-free treatment that can be used in conjunction with more traditional therapies. In order to improve general healing and wellbeing, it could be provided in addition to physical therapy, massage therapy, or psychotherapy.
- **Hospital settings:** As part of recovery programs for patients recuperating from surgeries or injuries, several hospitals and rehabilitation facilities are starting to investigate cold therapy. Cold plunges are used to control pain, inflammation, and swelling.

## 10.3 The Function of Education and Public Awareness

## The Need to Inform the Public About the Advantages and Dangers of Cold Plunging

Even if there are many advantages to cold plunging, it is crucial that the general public is aware of the hazards as well as the benefits:

- **Knowing the science**: Many people don't know the psychological and physiological processes that underlie cold treatment. Campaigns for public education can assist individuals learn about the advantages of cold exposure, how it works, and how to use it properly.
- The safe use of cold plunge should be emphasized in education programs so that people are aware of when and how to utilize cold treatment to prevent negative side effects.

## How Public Views of Cold Therapy Are Being Shaped by Scientific Communication

The public's perception of cold plunging is greatly influenced by scientific research and clinical trials:

- **Dissemination of research:** Universities, research organizations, and health care providers are increasingly sharing their findings via mainstream media, peer-reviewed publications, and wellness platforms. This promotes potential users to make educated decisions and helps to increase confidence in the efficacy of cold therapy.

- **Media and influencers:** Wellness influencers, fitness instructors, and celebrities that support cold treatment help to create favorable opinions about its advantages. To prevent false information, it is imperative that these recommendations are supported by reliable science.

## Initiatives to Encourage Conscientious and Knowledgeable Cold Plunging Use in Wellness Activities

It is the duty of the wellness community to guarantee the

safe and efficient application of cold therapy:

- **Certification and training:** Spas and wellness centers that provide cold plunging should make sure that their employees are well trained in cold treatment administration and client assessment.

- **Consumer guidelines:** The public should have access to clear guidelines and recommendations, such as details on ideal temperatures, session lengths, and the significance of a progressive adaptation to cold exposure.

The technique is set to play a big role in medical and wellness procedures as long as research into cold plunging and contrast therapy continues. Cold plunge has the potential to become a common treatment for a number of physical and mental health issues by increasing public awareness, incorporating cold therapy into healthcare, and furthering scientific research. This therapeutic approach will probably become a cornerstone of contemporary health and wellness programs through ongoing study and education.

# ABOUT THE AUTHOR

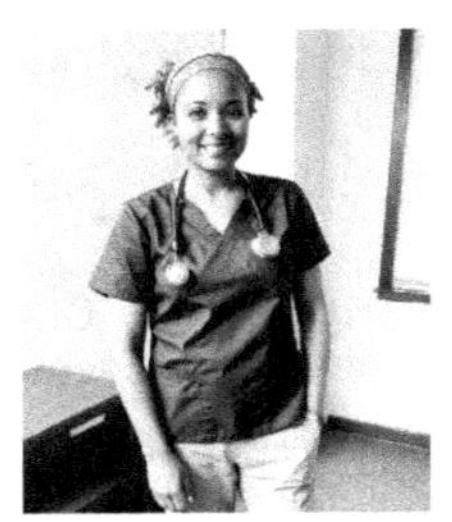 Harmony Royce is a dedicated healthcare worker who has a strong interest in holistic wellness. Harmony's extensive history in various aspects of health and wellness provides her with a wealth of knowledge and expertise that she can utilize in her writing and professional endeavors.

Harmony is a talented author who crafts thought-provoking books that inspire readers to have well-rounded, balanced lives. She writes about a variety of health-related topics, such as diet, exercise, mental health, and mindfulness. Her approachable writing style combines practical guidance with evidence-based research to make complex health concepts approachable and engaging for readers of all ages.

Harmony actively promotes the benefits of holistic health through writing, community workshops, and internet forums. Her mission is to educate and inspire people about the transformative power of self-care and healthy lifestyle choices.

9 798300 407513